The Power of Tai Chi

Master Shao Zhao-Ming

HB
HINKLER
BOOKS

Published by Hinkler Books Pty Ltd
45–55 Fairchild Street
Heatherton Victoria 3202 Australia
www.hinklerbooks.com

© Hinkler Books Pty Ltd 2009, 2010

Book cover design: Sam Grimmer and Mandi Cole
Editor: Kate Cuthbert
Art director: Leigh Ashforth
Photography: Ned Meldrum
Prepress: Graphic Print Group

Bamboo, butterfly and dragonfly © istockphoto.com
Cherry blossom with sunbeams © Peter Zelei/istockphoto.com
Chinese red landscape © Rolffimages/Dreamstime.com
Chinese traditional flower pattern © istockphoto.com
Human bones showing spine © Max Delson/istockphoto.com
Japanese style background © Peter Zelei/istockphoto.com
Mt. Huangshan © Zubin/istockphoto.com
Yin Yang symbol in a glow © istockphoto.com

Always do the warm-up exercises before attempting any individual exercises. It is
recommended that you check with your doctor or healthcare professional before
commencing any exercise. While every care has been taken in the preparation of
this material, the publishers and their respective employees or agents will not accept responsibility
for injury or damage occasioned to any person as a result of participation
in the activities described in this book.

ISBN: 978 1 7418 4469 6

Printed and bound in China

CONTENTS

INTRODUCTION   4

ABOUT TAI CHI   6
History   6
Different Styles of Tai Chi   7
Timeline of the Development of the Five Major
   Tai Chi Styles by the Founders   7
Martial Applications   9
Tai Chi Aids and Weapons   10
Tai Chi and You – Getting Better with Age   10

CHINESE PHILOSOPHY
AND TAI CHI   12
Origins of Chinese Philosophy   12
The Yin Yang Symbol   12
The Meaning of Tai Chi   13

THE CONCEPT OF QI   14
Qi   14
Dan Tian   14

BREATHING   16

BENEFITS OF TAI CHI   18
Tai Chi Physical Benefits in the Western Context   18
Tai Chi in the Context of Traditional Chinese
   Medicine (TCM)   19

GETTING STARTED   19

WARM-UP EXERCISES   20
1   Arms – Swinging   21
2   Shoulders – Rotating   21
3   Wrists – Rotating and Stretching   22
4   Neck – Stretching Forwards and Backwards   22
5   Neck – Stretching Sides   23
6   Lower Back and Hips   23
7   Knees   24
8   Ankles   25

QI GONG EXERCISES   26
Lao Gong   27
Bai Hui   28
Ming Men   29
Qi Gong Exercise 1 – Rooster Crowing in
   the Morning   30
Qi Gong Exercise 2 – Boosting the Qi   32

TAI CHI BASICS   36
Tai Chi Posture   37
Coordination of Handwork and Footwork   37
Horse Stance   38
Bow Stance   38
Empty Stance   38
Stepping Forwards and Backwards   39
Stepping Out to the Corner   40

TAI CHI 8 FORM   42
Raising Hands   43
Repulse Monkey   44
Brush Knee   45
Parting the Horse's Mane   46
Cloud Hands (without stepping)   47
Golden Rooster Stands on One Leg   47
Jade Lady   48
Press and Push   49
Cross Hands   51
Closing   51

COOLING DOWN EXERCISES   52
Relaxation Massage   52
Returning Qi to the Origin   55

TAI CHI STANDING
MEDITATION   56
Meditative Sequence   58

CONCLUSION   61

ABOUT THE AUTHOR   62

ACKNOWLEDGEMENTS   64

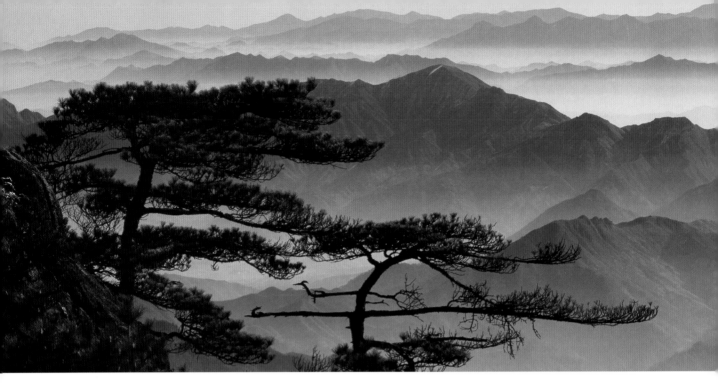

INTRODUCTION

Tai Chi has experienced a phenomenal increase in popularity in recent years, largely due to a growing public awareness of its many health benefits and versatility. As Western science gradually comes to realise the many positive benefits of Tai Chi, more and more people are taking it up. At the same time, there is a rising number of health professionals recognising the unique benefits of Tai Chi, and advising their clients to use this exercise system to improve both their physical and mental health. Tai Chi is low impact, suitable for all age groups and very convenient – you can practise indoors or outdoors, with or without equipment and alone or in groups!

Due to its long history, many styles of Tai Chi have evolved. No matter which style of Tai Chi people practise, one thing is certain – we can all benefit from the regular practice of this marvellous exercise system.

In this book, we will explore:

- **Tai Chi philosophy** – An understanding of the philosophy behind Tai Chi will help you understand techniques and grasp more advanced concepts.

- **Warm-up exercises** – Warming up before Tai Chi helps to enhance its effectiveness and reduce the risk of any strains or injuries. Warm ups also

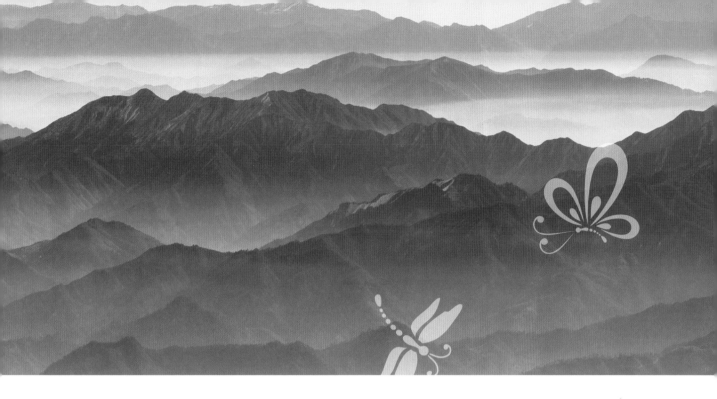

help maintain mobility and flexibility, which are important components of good physical health.

- **Qi Gong exercises** – Qi Gong exercises in this book can be used as part of your Tai Chi practice to enhance its effectiveness, or they can be practised on their own at any time to help cultivate qi and maintain good health. Use Qi Gong exercises to give yourself a boost of energy at anytime.

- **Tai Chi basics** – It is important to practise Tai Chi correctly in order to benefit as much as possible. A good grasp of the basics is key.

- **Tai Chi 8 form** – This short Tai Chi form is good for general relaxation and to maintain mobility and physical health. It is a great foundation for further Tai Chi practice in the future.

- **Cooling down exercises** – Use these anytime you want to unwind and calm down, including after a Tai Chi practice.

- **Tai Chi standing meditation** – This exercise is a gem for the cultivation of qi, in particular the Dan Tian qi, and to enhance and maintain good health. It is indispensable for advanced Tai Chi practice.

Application of these specially designed exercises and standing meditation will help you develop and increase Dan Tian qi directly and instantly. This is the essence of the Chinese healing art of Tai Chi.

ABOUT TAI CHI

HISTORY

From the chaos of war and martial conflict, a gentle system of exercise with strong benefits for humankind was developed. Such extremities, symbolised by the Yin Yang symbol, represent the basic philosophy of the martial art, which evolved into the exercise system we now call Tai Chi. Tai Chi is also known as 'Tai Chi Chuan', 'Shadow Boxing', 'Taiji' and 'Taijiquan'.

The beginnings of Tai Chi have long been a topic of debate. Popular belief has the birth of Tai Chi as early as the eighth century, while many attribute a Taoist priest, Zhang Shan Feng, as the founder of Tai Chi in the fifteenth century. Research done in the 1930s by martial arts Master and historian Tang Hao and others suggests that Tai Chi originated in the 1660s, and was developed by Chen Wang Ting of the Henan province in China. Chen was the chief of civil troops defending Wen County in the Henan province. He was skilled in martial arts, and his techniques were passed from generation to generation. Over time, his form of martial arts developed into many different styles, characterised by the people who learned and spread the skill.

These findings are supported by evidence gathered in 2007 by a team of martial arts experts, historians and folklore experts commissioned by the Chinese Folklore Association. This team performed extensive research and analysis, and concluded that Wen County is the birthplace of Tai Chi.

The five major styles of Tai Chi are Chen, Yang, Wu, Woo and Sun. This book will introduce you to Yang-style Tai Chi because of its relatively simple principles, movements and posture, which makes it a great first step for beginners.

DIFFERENT STYLES OF TAI CHI

The different styles of Tai Chi are characterised by their principles, movements and application. To give you an idea, let's have a look at the characteristics of the five major styles:

- **Chen** – Movements emphasise softness with hardness. Movements are obviously circular with much spiralling. The body leads the hands, and the waist is the axis. Chen-style Tai Chi is more suitable for advanced practitioners, and is a deceivingly powerful martial art.

- **Yang** – Movements are larger and more extended. The posture is upright and full. The pace is gentle, slow and continuous, with connections between movements gentle and coherent. The force of movements is internal with tenderness and fierceness. Yang is very popular with Tai Chi beginners.

- **Wu** – Movements and postures are compact and simple. The momentum is delicate and centred with awareness; the process of movement is consistent and rhythmic with many closings and openings. The pace is comfortable, and the mind's focus is beyond the movements. Hands are kept upward. Each hand is concerned with movements of its own side of the body.

- **Woo** – Movements are moderately wide, compact and balanced; the momentum is elegant and refined, delicate and agile. Connection between movements is fine and smooth, natural and relaxed; the speed is constant and continuous without intervals. There is an emphasis on softness.

- **Sun** – Movements are compact. This style is characterised by a high and upright posture and lively footwork. Sun style is the youngest of the five major styles of Tai Chi.

TIMELINE OF THE DEVELOPMENT OF THE FIVE MAJOR TAI CHI STYLES BY THE FOUNDERS

Chen Style	Yang Style	Wu Style	Woo Style		Sun Style
by Chen Wang Ting	*by Yang Lu Chan*	*by Wu Yu Xiang*	*by Quan You & Wu Jian Qua*		*by Sun Lu Tang*
1660s	*1799–1872*	*1812–1880*	*1834–1902*	*1870–1942*	*1861–1932*

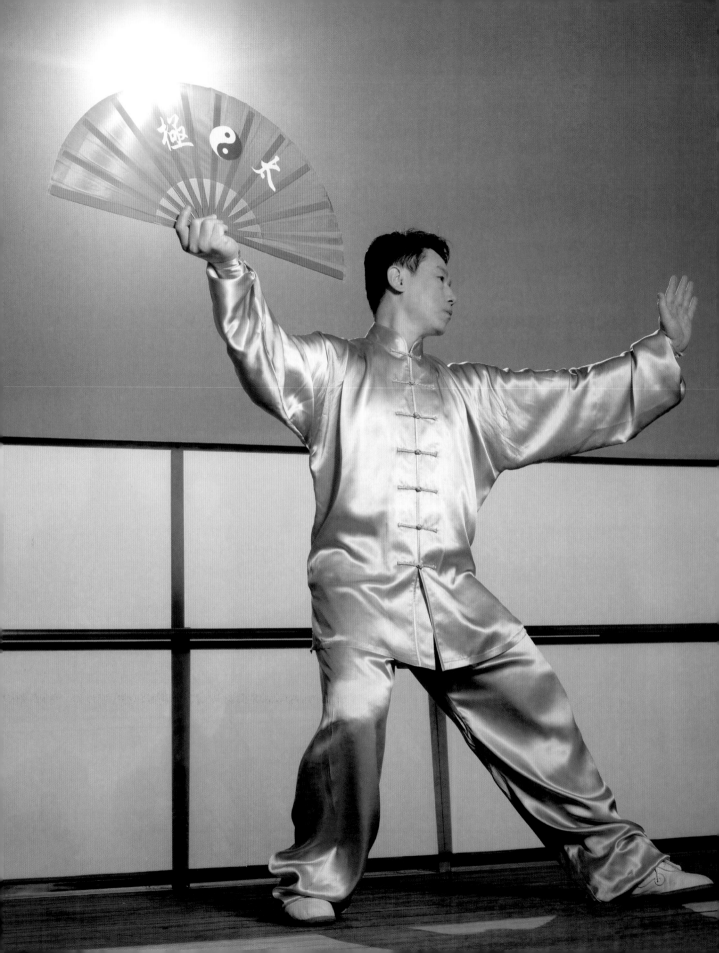

MARTIAL APPLICATIONS

Without doubt, the original system of Tai Chi was developed as a form of martial arts. It was only with time that the health benefits of Tai Chi became apparent, resulting in a following of practitioners who practise solely for health reasons. This does not overshadow the fact that there remain practitioners whose interest is to learn Tai Chi as a form of martial arts.

Practising Tai Chi as a martial art requires great commitment from the practitioner. He or she must have solid understanding of the principles, philosophies, culture and application of Tai Chi in a martial context. The skill-level of the Tai Chi martial artist needs to be relatively advanced in order to properly apply Tai Chi techniques in a martial context. Tai Chi is classified as an internal branch of martial arts, meaning that it is a martial art concerned with internal power. Therefore, the Tai Chi martial artist must develop inner strength and cultivate qi.

As an exercise system, Tai Chi movements are graceful and gentle, often described as moving meditation. As a martial art, Tai Chi is deceivingly powerful. Tai Chi martial art techniques are characterised by the use of leverage to neutralise or initiate attacks. The leverage is achieved by coordinating a combination of relaxed movements and the strategic use of joints and inner strength to redirect an opponent's force.

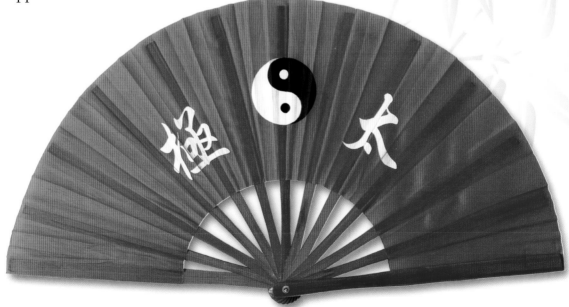

TAI CHI AIDS AND WEAPONS

There are many aids and training weapons that can be used in further Tai Chi study. These are especially interesting and can add a very enjoyable aspect to your Tai Chi practice. Common aids include the Tai Chi ball and Tai Chi ruler, both of which help to improve technique, awareness and cultivation of qi.

Popular training weapons in Tai Chi include the sword, fan, pole (also known as staff/cudgel) and spear. Tai Chi weapons have been specially developed to be non-threatening when used properly. For example, the Tai Chi sword is either a blunt, hollow telescopic device that extends out to resemble a sword, or a device with a sword handle and thin, very flexible non-sharpened blade. Aids and training weapons can be easily purchased from most martial art supply shops or the internet. Some countries may have guidelines about the purchase, import and use of training weapons in public places.

TAI CHI AND YOU – GETTING BETTER WITH AGE

One thing distinguishes Tai Chi from most other forms of exercise – age is no barrier and you will only get better and better with practice. By now, you will realise that Tai Chi can be enjoyed as a regular, simple exercise program, or studied in-depth and practised for a lifetime. The beauty is that no matter how far you decide to take your Tai Chi practice, you stand to gain a lifetime of benefits!

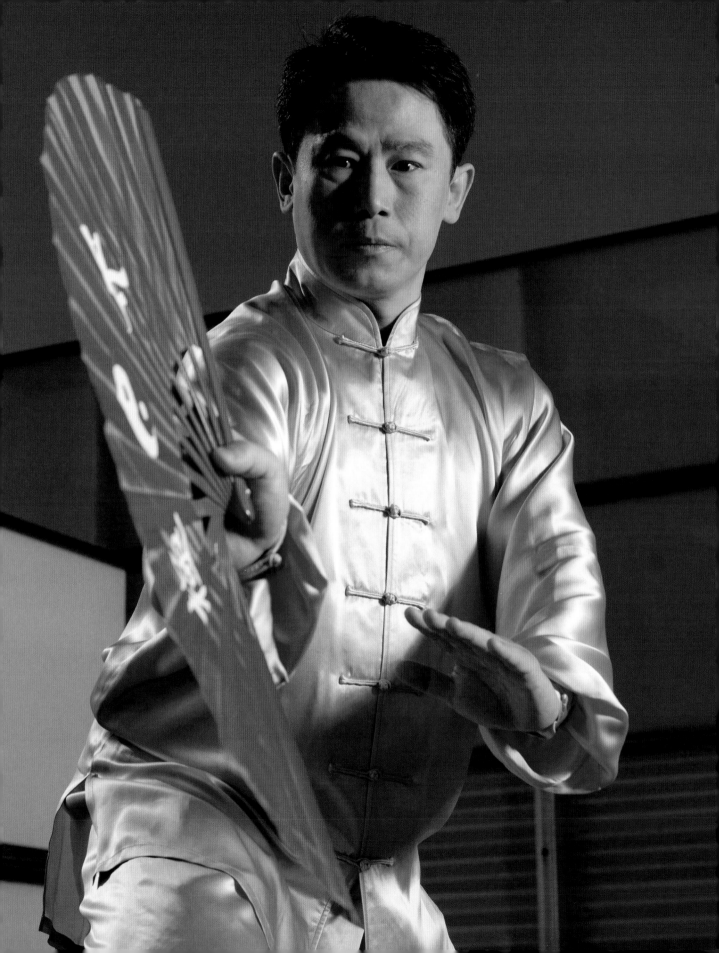

CHINESE PHILOSOPHY AND TAI CHI

ORIGINS OF CHINESE PHILOSOPHY

The origins of Chinese philosophy are often traced back to an ancient Chinese text, known as the I-Ching (Book of Changes). The I-Ching contains a set of predictions or outcomes represented by 64 hexagrams ('gua' in Chinese). The text is traditionally believed to date back as far as 2800 BC, and its contents developed from ancient Chinese philosophy and cosmology or understanding of the natural phenomena of our universe. The cosmology centres on the ideas of:

- the interplay and balance of opposites (known commonly as Yin and Yang)
- the natural evolution of events as a process
- the inevitability of change, which must be accepted.

THE YIN YANG SYMBOL

Yang is the male, light, warm, extrovert, active aspect, shown as the white portions.

Yin is the female, dark, cold, introvert, passive side of life, indicated by the black portions.

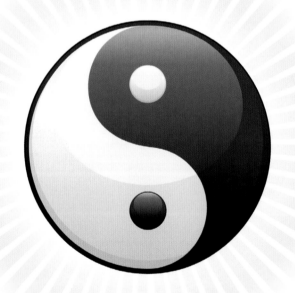

The Yin Yang symbol represents the natural interplay of the dual forces of Yin and Yang (or opposing forces) in our universe.

The dot in each Yin and Yang area indicate that Yin contains the seeds of Yang, and Yang contains the seeds of Yin – the forces always coexist, and one does not exist without the other. As an example, Yang is like man, Yin is like woman. Yang cannot exist without Yin. Yin cannot give birth without Yang.

Everything in the universe (shown as the outer complete circle) consists of both Yin and Yang. The forces are opposites, but complementary so long as they are balanced. Yin and Yang forces must be in balance for harmony to exist and for all things to function properly. When the forces are out of balance, conflict arises and proper function ceases.

The curved lines indicate that nothing is absolute, for whatever reaches the extreme has already started towards its opposite. The underlying principle is complete balance and harmony.

THE MEANING OF TAI CHI

Literally translated from Chinese, Tai Chi means 'Supreme Ultimate'. It is a simultaneous state of infinite potential and of absolute, in line with the principles of Yin and Yang. The modern exercise system of Tai Chi is more accurately known in China as Taijiquan (or Tai Chi Chuan), meaning 'Supreme Ultimate Boxing'. Tai Chi Chuan theory and practice embraces many of the principles of Chinese philosophy.

In the context of Tai Chi Chuan, the human body is a universe, and all its parts are exercised in balance to enable harmony in function. The following table can give you an idea of what represents Yin and Yang in the context of Tai Chi Chuan:

Yin	Yang
Inhale	Exhale
Lower body	Upper body
Front of body	Back of body
Right side of body	Left side of body
Inside of limbs	Outside of limbs
Step forwards	Retreat
Stillness	Motion

THE CONCEPT OF QI

QI

Qi (also known as chi) can be described as personal bioenergy in our body. Tai Chi and Qi Gong are ancient Chinese exercises used to promote qi for self-healing and wellbeing. Traditional Chinese medicine is based on the belief that the body consists of a network of energy channels called meridians. Qi, or bioenergy, travels along these meridians to bring vital energy to the body and organs. Illness is associated with a weak, interrupted or blocked flow of qi. It is not uncommon for knowledgeable doctors of Chinese medicine to prescribe Tai Chi or Qi Gong exercises to help improve some health conditions. The cultivation and healthy flow of qi is essential for a longer, healthier life, and for faster recovery from illness and injury.

DAN TIAN

Literally translated from Chinese, Dan Tian means 'Elixir Field' – it is where qi and the body's essence are stored and cultivated. In Chinese medicine and martial arts, it is understood that our upper body has three Dan Tians.

Basic functions of the three Dan Tians:

- **Upper Dan Tian** – This field stores and cultivates the mind's spirit.
- **Middle Dan Tian** – This field stores, gathers and purifies the qi. Middle Dan Tian is concerned with post-natal qi.
- **Lower Dan Tian** – This field stores and cultivates the original qi and essence of the body. Original qi refers to the qi one is born with. Lower Dan Tian is therefore concerned with pre-natal qi.

Tai Chi and Qi Gong exercises can be viewed as post-natal techniques that help to promote optimum function of the Dan Tians, thereby maintaining a healthy level of qi in the body. Tai Chi at a beginner level is mainly concerned with the Lower Dan Tian – therefore in this book we will focus on the Lower Dan Tian.

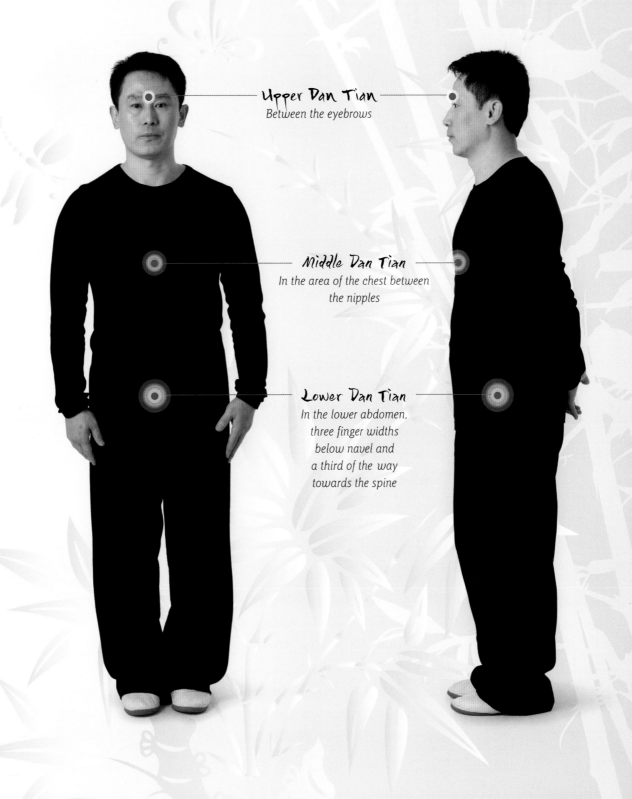

Upper Dan Tian
Between the eyebrows

Middle Dan Tian
*In the area of the chest between
the nipples*

Lower Dan Tian
*In the lower abdomen,
three finger widths
below navel and
a third of the way
towards the spine*

BREATHING

There are different ways of breathing:

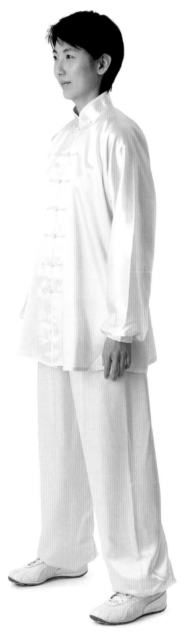

- **Natural breathing** – this is the way most people breathe. We breathe in and out through the nose, with chest/lungs inflating and deflating accordingly. In this type of breathing, the lungs are expanded and contracted by the muscles of the chest. For Tai Chi beginners, it is most appropriate to start with natural breathing.

- **Natural abdominal breathing** – this is far more effective than natural breathing. As babies, this is how we instinctively breathe after birth, before mysteriously changing to natural breathing in later childhood. In this type of breathing, the lungs are expanded and contracted by the muscles of the diaphragm and abdomen rather than the chest muscles. Breathe in deeply with the intention of filling up the lungs from the bottom up, causing the lower abdomen to expand, progressing to the mid-abdomen and slightly into the chest. Breathe out slowly and gradually, causing deflation to occur from the mid-abdomen to the lower abdomen. It is best to progress from natural breathing to abdominal breathing after some practice, as it will greatly enhance the health benefits of Tai Chi and Qi Gong.

- **Reverse abdominal breathing** – the abdomen is drawn in when breathing in, and expanded when breathing out. In this type of breathing, the diaphragm and abdominal muscles are used. It is most suitable for advanced practitioners, who can use this form of breathing to help direct qi within the body to increase inner strength and power. This type of breathing should initially be attempted under the supervision of an experienced instructor.

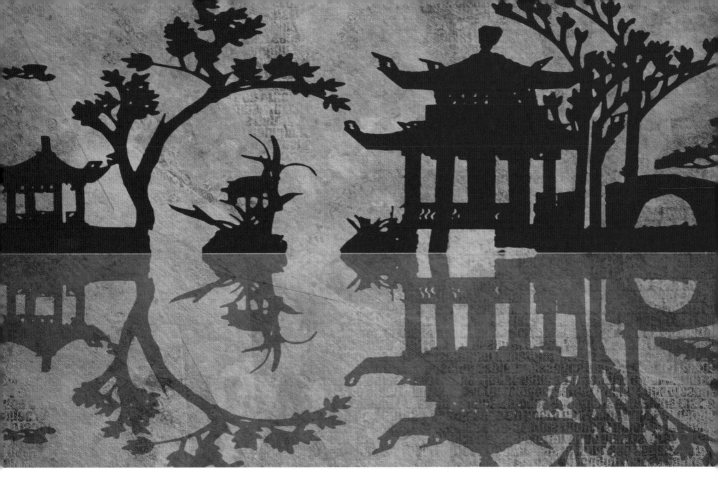

For the purpose of this book, start with natural breathing when you first attempt the exercises, then progress to natural abdominal breathing once you become more familiar with the movements. To do natural abdominal breathing effectively, follow these steps:

1. Breathe in while focusing the mind, starting from the lower abdomen, progressing upwards to the mid-abdomen and finally into the chest.

2. Breathe out while focusing the mind, starting from the chest, progressing down to the mid-abdomen and finally into the lower abdomen.

Note

Throughout this book, you will note that the instructions for some steps commence with 'breathe in' or 'breathe out'. It is vital that you try to coordinate the breathing in/out for the entire duration of that particular step. Avoid holding your breath while finishing off the movement of that step. It may take some time to get the coordination and timing right, but you feel much better when your breathing is correctly timed with your movements.

BENEFITS OF TAI CHI

Due to the completeness of Tai Chi, the benefits are many and varied. The health and physical condition of every individual is unique, however, and the benefits each individual experiences will be dependent on this. The quality and quantity of Tai Chi practice will also play a part. Commonly, people who practise Tai Chi regularly may experience improvements in various conditions including stress relief, arthritis, diabetes, high blood pressure, heart health, chronic pain, insomnia and digestive problems. It is also common for practitioners to experience improvement in general health, coordination, balance, strength and flexibility, self-awareness and concentration.

TAI CHI PHYSICAL BENEFITS IN THE WESTERN CONTEXT

Correct body posture aligns the spine and:
- releases tension and pressure caused by bad posture
- reduces stress on back
- improves digestion.

Whole-body movements are diverse and varied, involving gentle weight bearing and use of all joints. Regular practice:
- increases joint mobility, aiding arthritis, chronic pain and similar conditions
- maintains and increases muscles and ligament strength
- improves coordination
- increases and maintains bone density
- massages internal organs by increasing the flow of bodily fluids and circulation, improving functions
- aids recovery from accidents and surgery.

Movements are controlled and deliberately slow which:
- looks deceivingly easy, but is highly effective in building and maintaining muscle and tendon strength with proper practice
- builds balance
- maintains and can improve cardiovascular health and stamina.

Tai Chi in the Context of Traditional Chinese Medicine (TCM)

TCM recognises and treats each individual as a whole system (or universe), taking into consideration all aspects of the mind, body and soul. Tai Chi:

- improves physical health through its specially designed whole-body movements and breathing methods
- cultivates and stimulates energy flow (qi/bioenergy)
- promotes spiritual, emotional and mental health through its gentle, meditative exercises that help to relax, clear and clarify the mind.

Tai Chi and Qi Gong philosophies are closely linked with the universal principles of Yin and Yang. The philosophies are applicable in everyday life.

It is important to bear in mind that Tai Chi needs to be practised correctly and regularly in order to maximise benefits for the practitioner.

GETTING STARTED

Getting started in Tai Chi is easy. All you really need is a safe, relatively comfortable environment and loose, comfortable clothing. As a guide, the ideal environment may have the following features:

- good ventilation
- comfortable, relaxing atmosphere
- comfortable temperature
- access to relaxing music, if desired.

Place yourself in a calm, relaxed frame of mind and focus on yourself.

The Tai Chi movements in this book are very simple and easy to follow. Each movement is repeated on both the right and left sides of the body. You can practise each movement as many times as you like. The next movement follows in direct sequence from the previous movement, unless otherwise stated, so be sure to stay in your finishing position to start the next movement. As you learn the moves, you will find that you will be able to flow through your Tai Chi practice with ease and grace.

Warm-up Exercises

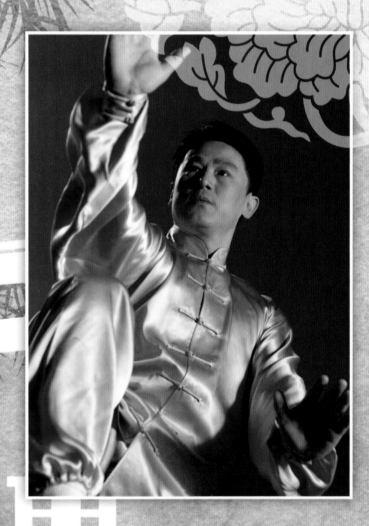

ARMS – SWINGING　左右甩臂

This exercise loosens up the tensions in the shoulder, arms and back, especially for those who spend a lot of time working in front of computers, or have some stiffness in these joints.

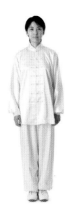 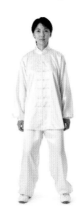 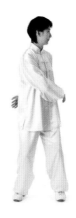

1 Stand with feet shoulder width apart, knees slightly bent and head upright. Relax your arms, lower back and hips.

2 Swing your arms side to side, hands gently patting your lower back and the sides of your waist.

3 Turn your upper body and head as you swing your arms.

SHOULDERS – ROTATING　前后转肩

This exercise loosens the tensions of the shoulders and shoulder blades, increases circulation to the neck and relieves discomfort of the upper back.

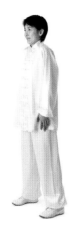 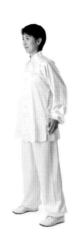 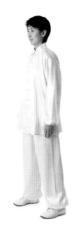 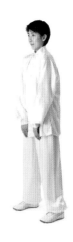

1 Lift your shoulders up, roll backwards and down, then forwards and up. Repeat several times.

2 Reverse direction by lifting your shoulders up and rolling them forwards and down, then backwards and up. Repeat several times.

WRISTS – ROTATING AND STRETCHING
旋转，牵拉碗关节

Stretching the tendons around the wrists will help relieve the tension
of repetitive stress injuries and carpal tunnel syndrome.

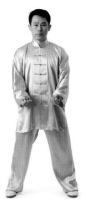
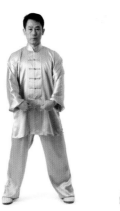
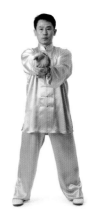

1 Gently form your hands into fists and
rotate your wrists inwards several times,
then reverse direction and rotate outwards.

2 To stretch your wrists and forearm,
outstretch one arm and gently pull back
the fingers of that hand for a few seconds.
Repeat on the other side.

3 Relax your hands and
arms and gently shake
a few times.

NECK – STRETCHING FORWARDS AND BACKWARDS
前后牵拉颈项

This exercise loosens muscle tensions of the neck and helps mobility
in the neck joints. Using your hands to support your neck will help avoid
straining any muscles and prevent any injuries for those with neck disorders.

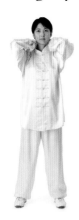
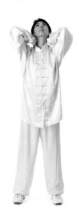
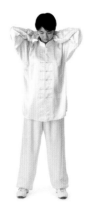
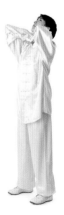

1 Place your hands
around your neck,
fingers supporting
the back of neck.

2 Pressing the back of your neck,
gently bring your head upwards
(going only as far as you are
comfortable).

3 Keep your hands supporting your neck
and gently bring your head forwards and
look downwards (going only as far as
you are comfortable).

4 Repeat
several times.

NECK – STRETCHING SIDES 左右牵拉颈项

This exercise helps loosen muscle tensions in the neck, increase mobility of the neck joints and get more stretch along the side of the neck.

1 Place one hand on your opposite shoulder, press down gently and tilt your head to the opposite direction (going only as far as you are comfortable).

2 Repeat for other side, and stretch both sides several times.

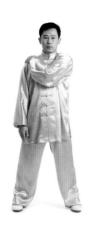
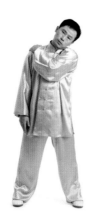
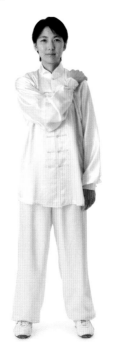
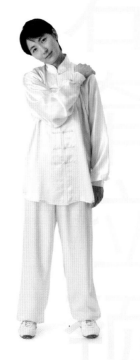

LOWER BACK AND HIPS 旋转腰胯

Relieve stiffness of the lower back and hips by gently stretching these joints.

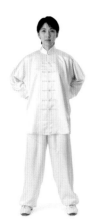
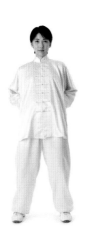
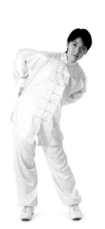
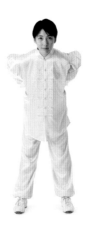
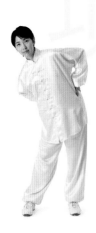

1 Place your palms against your lower back and hips for support, and rotate clockwise several times.

2 Repeat in an anticlockwise direction several times.

KNEES   旋转膝关节

This exercise stretches the ligaments around the knee, to prevent strain.

1 Bring your feet in slightly, leaving about two fists' distance between your feet.

2 Place your hands on your knees, and massage around the front and back of your knees, shins and calves.

3 With your hands on your knees, bend your knees and separate them outwards in a circular motion several times.

4 Reverse direction and rotate your knees inwards in a circular motion several times.

5 Bend your knees and straighten while standing upright.

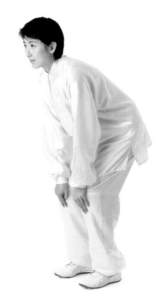
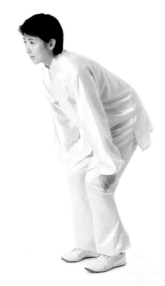
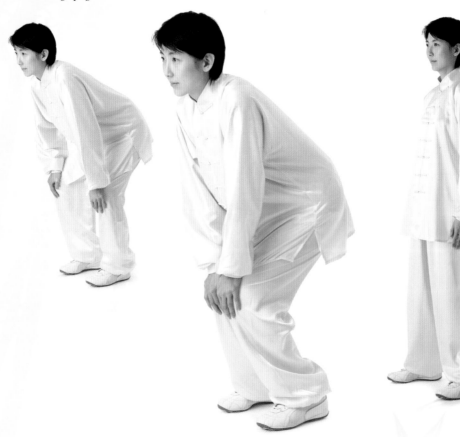

ANKLES 旋转踝关节

Stretch the ligaments and tendons around the ankles to help prevent strain.

1 Shift weight to the left and lift your right foot in front of you.

2 Point your toes up, then down, and rotate clockwise a few times, then rotate anticlockwise a few times.

3 Repeat on the other side.

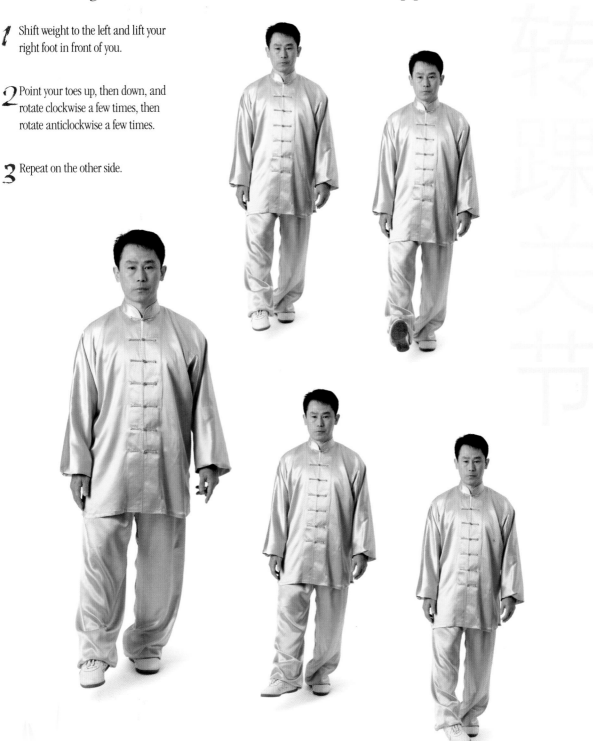

Qi Gong Exercises

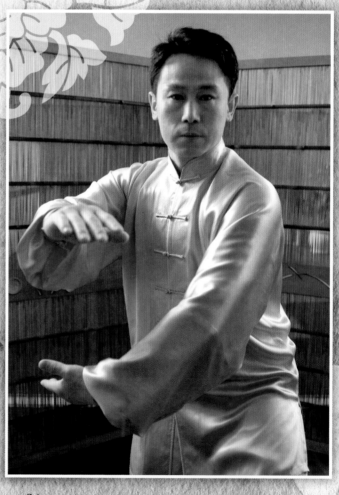

The benefits of Tai Chi can be increased by doing some Qi Gong exercises beforehand, to stimulate the flow of qi. To achieve this, we need to know a little about some important pressure points. It is best to do Qi Gong exercises after the warm-ups but before commencing Tai Chi.

Some important pressure points:

LAO GONG 劳宫

Literally translated, 'Lao Gong' means 'Labour Palace'. This pressure point complements and nurtures the heart. Appropriate stimulation can help with cardiac disorders, mental stress and fatigue. In the context of qi, this pressure point is regarded as the window of the human body. Stimulating this point during Qi Gong and before Tai Chi helps to get the qi flowing, aids the hands in absorbing qi from nature and increases sensitivity of qi between the hands and body.

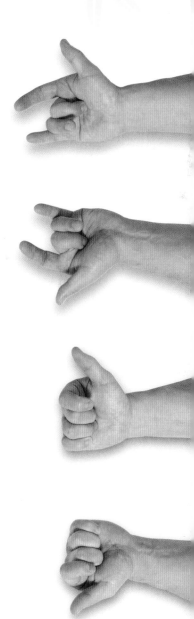

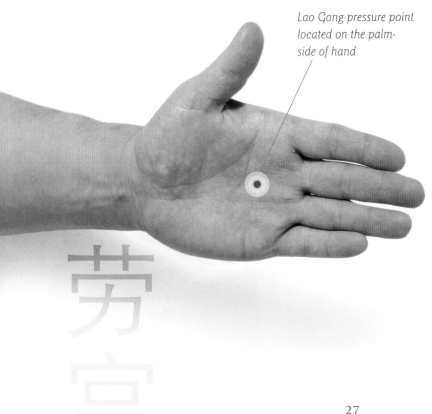

Lao Gong pressure point located on the palm-side of hand

劳宫

Bai Hui 百会

Literally translated, Bai Hui means 'Gathering of Hundreds'. It refers to the point where Yang energy is concentrated. Appropriate stimulation of this point can help with dizziness, headaches, memory, insomnia, faintness, unbalanced blood pressure, blurred vision, nasal obstruction, prolapse of the rectum or uterus, mental disorders and brain disease. In the context of qi, this pressure point can help to straighten one's posture, sink down the shoulder joints and relax the chest and abdominals, thus aiding the smooth flow of qi.

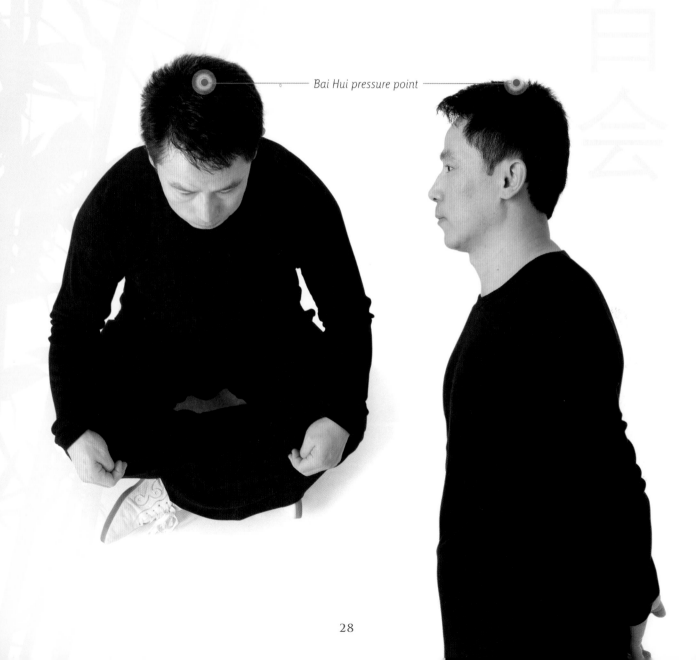

Bai Hui pressure point

MING MEN 命门

Literally translated, Ming Men means 'Gate of Life'. It is concerned with delivering fire/warm energy to the kidneys, which nourish other organs in the body. In Chinese medicine, the kidneys are considered to be the root of pre-natal energy. Ming Men is located on the back, directly on the vertebrae and horizontally aligned with the navel. Appropriate stimulation of this point can assist in the treatment of diseases of the genital system including impotence, ejaculatory problems, irregular menstruation, chronic diarrhoea and back/spinal aches.

When doing Tai Chi forms and Standing Meditation, this pressure point should be consciously pushed backwards, by focusing your mind. This will sink the qi to the Lower Dan Tian, relaxing the lower back, and allow your movements to originate from the waist and involve the Lower Dan Tian. This point is the source of our Tai Chi movement.

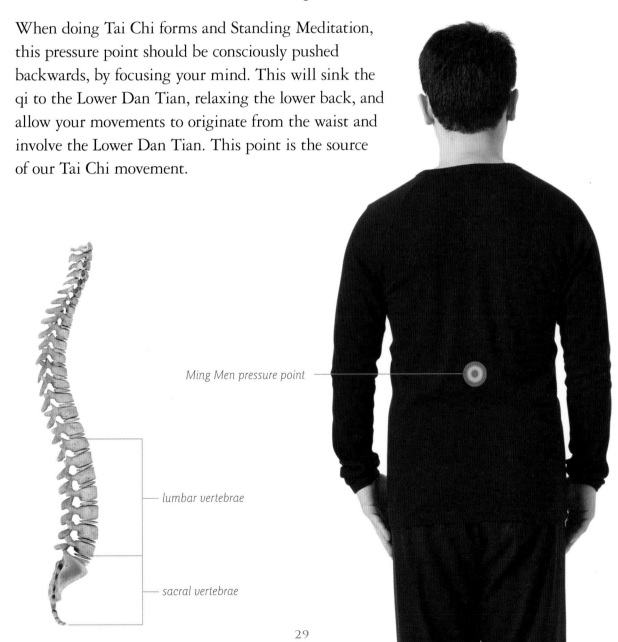

Ming Men pressure point

lumbar vertebrae

sacral vertebrae

QI GONG EXERCISE 1 – ROOSTER CROWING IN THE MORNING 金鸡报晓

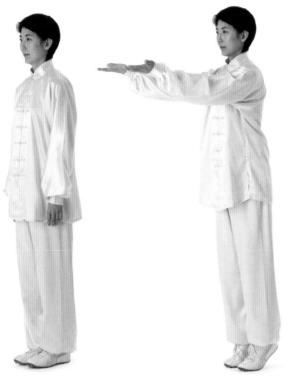

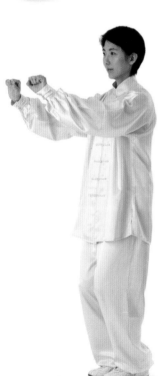

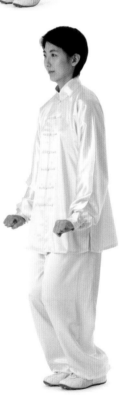

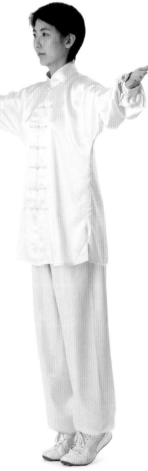

1 Stand with your feet together. Focus on using the Bai Hui pressure point to lead your head upwards and relax your entire body.

2 Breathe in and bring your hands up to the front at shoulder height, palms facing up, lifting your heels.

3 Breathe out while turning your palms face down, bending both middle fingers in to press the Lao Gong pressure point. Simultaneously drop your arms and heels down, keeping knees slightly bent.

4 Breathe in and raise your hands up from side to shoulder height, palms facing up and heels lifted.

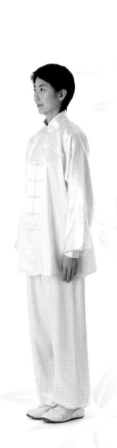

5 Breathe out and turn your palms face down, bend both middle fingers in to press the Lao Gong pressure point, and simultaneously drop arms and heels down, keeping knees slightly bent.

6 Breathe in and push palms backwards, lifting heels up.

7 Breathe out and bend both middle fingers in to press the Lao Gong pressure point, dropping arms and heels down, keeping knees slightly bent.

8 Repeat several times.

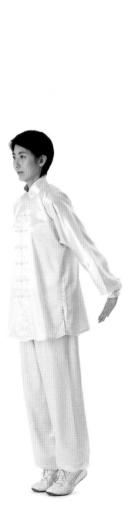

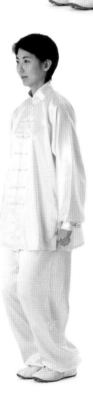

QI GONG EXERCISE 2 – BOOSTING THE QI 催气法

This exercise helps to develop good posture, which is an important element of Tai Chi. It also strengthens the thighs and knees. Standing up and down while opening and closing palms towards each other helps to increase the sensation of qi and the gathering of qi through the Lao Gong pressure points.

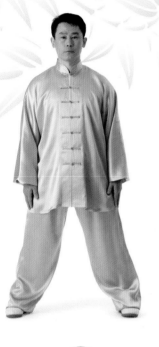

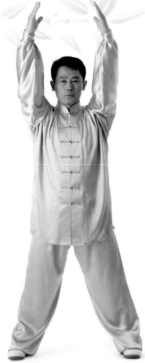

1 Stand with your feet shoulder width apart, arms beside your body and focus on using the Bai Hui pressure point to lead your head upwards.

2 Turning your palms up, raise your hands from the side of your body to above your head.

3 Lower your arms into the 'holding a ball' position, level at your throat, knees slightly bent. Maintain this posture for a few minutes or as long as you are comfortable.

4 Bend both middle fingers in to press the palms' Lao Gong pressure points while remaining in this posture. Release pressing and breathe in, separating your palms to shoulder width and standing up slowly. Keep your palms and each set of fingertips pointed at each other.

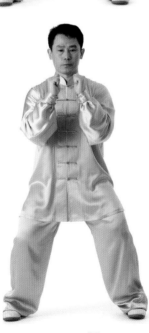

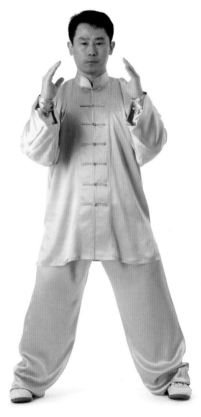

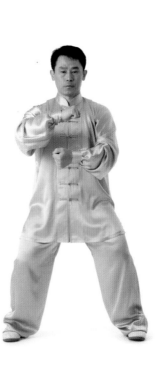

5 Breathe out and close your palms towards each other, while bending your knees slightly. Keep your palms and each set of fingertips pointed at each other into the 'holding a ball' position.

6 Repeat opening/closing your palms motion a few more times.

7 Bend both middle fingers in to press your palms' Lao Gong pressure points, while turning both palms to face each other, right hand on top.

8 Release pressing and breathe in. Open hands vertically (top hand to just above the head, bottom hand at groin height) and stand up slowly.

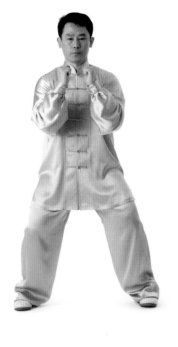

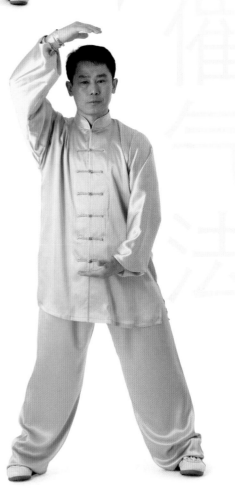

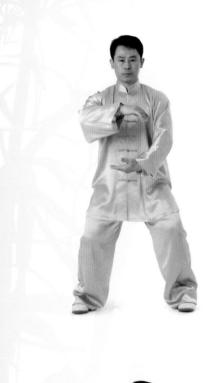

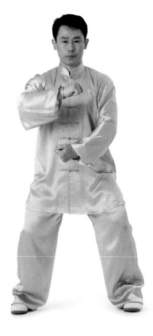

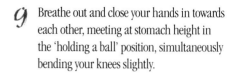

9 Breathe out and close your hands in towards each other, meeting at stomach height in the 'holding a ball' position, simultaneously bending your knees slightly.

10 Repeat opening/closing a few more times.

11 Bending both middle fingers in to press your palms' Lao Gong pressure points, rotate your hands to swap the positions of top and bottom hands .

12 Release pressing and breathe in, opening your hands vertically (top hand to just above the head, bottom hand at groin height) and stand up slowly.

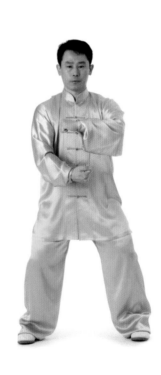

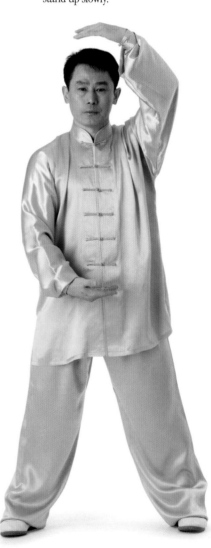

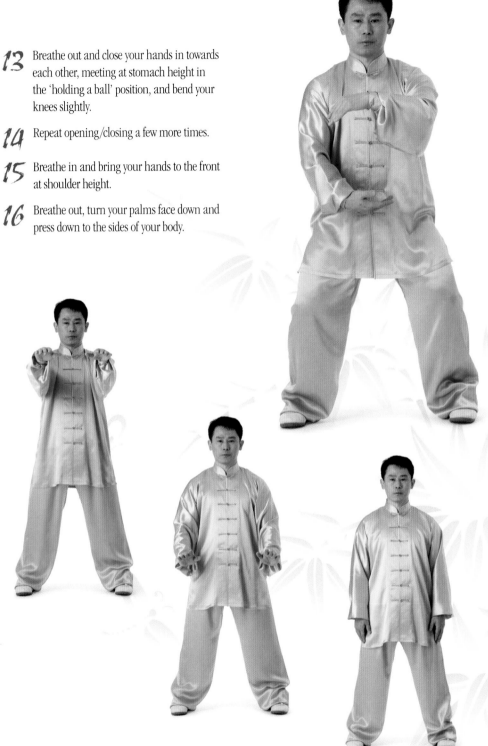

13 Breathe out and close your hands in towards each other, meeting at stomach height in the 'holding a ball' position, and bend your knees slightly.

14 Repeat opening/closing a few more times.

15 Breathe in and bring your hands to the front at shoulder height.

16 Breathe out, turn your palms face down and press down to the sides of your body.

Notes

During this exercise, you should keep check the tongue gently touching the top of your mouth's palate. Doing this will help connect the Governor and Conception Meridians, helping the flow of qi. It also generates saliva, which is considered an important body fluid in Chinese medicine, nourishing the organs, reducing stress and helping to centre your mind.

Tai Chi Basics

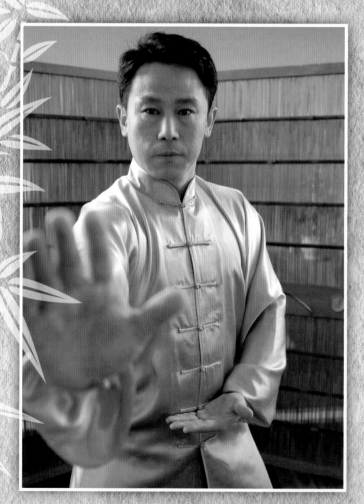

Learning the basics will help you gain the most from your Tai Chi practice.

TAI CHI POSTURE

The principles for correct Tai Chi posture apply for all Tai Chi movements. Correct Tai Chi posture is a key element to:

* getting your Tai Chi movements correct

* optimising the flow of qi

* gaining the maximum benefits from Tai Chi.

In order to achieve correct Tai Chi posture, raise the head up by focusing on using the Bai Hui pressure point to lead your head upwards, draw the chest in slightly, relax the lower back by consciously pushing the Ming Men pressure point backwards, sink the shoulders down, drop the elbows and tuck in the pelvis.

With correct Tai Chi posture, you will notice that the spine and back are straightened and the natural arch is reduced. Natural abdominal breathing should occur quite naturally.

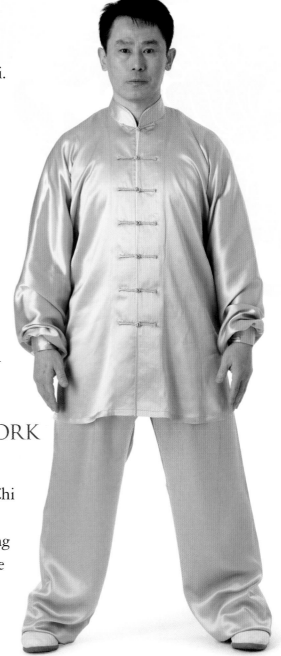

COORDINATION OF HANDWORK AND FOOTWORK

One of the major principles of Yang-style Tai Chi is that the handwork and footwork of each movement starts and finishes together. Applying this principle will help you coordinate and time your movements smoothly.

HORSE STANCE 马步

Horse Stance is used in many different martial arts. The Tai Chi Horse Stance is considered a relatively high stance.

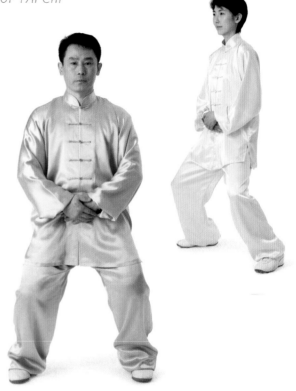

1 Stand with your feet shoulder width apart and your head upright. For the purpose of learning the Horse Stance, place your hands over the lower Dan Tian area.

2 Sink your body down by relaxing your lower back and hips and bend your knees outwards, keeping your feet slightly open. When you look down to your feet, you should notice that the angle of your feet is aligned with your thighs.

Notes

When you are in Horse Stance, you should always try to consciously push the Ming Men pressure point backwards. This will sink the qi down to the Lower Dan Tian and stretch the spine, thus aiding the smooth flow of qi.

BOW STANCE 弓步

1 Stand with one leg forwards, knee bent.

2 Keep your back leg's knee slightly bent as well, to allow your hip to sink downwards.

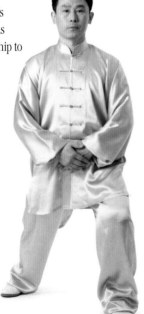

EMPTY STANCE 虚步

1 Stand with one leg about one step forwards – front foot is either on toes or heel, depending on the movement/posture.

2 Keep back leg's knee bent – back leg carries most of the body weight.

Notes

This stance on the heel is used in transitions of some movements in the Tai Chi 8 form.

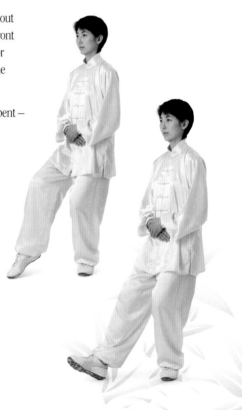

This is the basic stepping for Tai Chi 8 form in this book.

STEPPING FORWARDS AND BACKWARDS
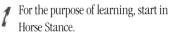

1 For the purpose of learning, start in Horse Stance.

2 Shift weight to the left, stepping out with your right heel and transferring your weight forwards, forming Bow Stance.

3 Shift your weight backwards, lift your front foot and step back in. Shift your weight to the right.

4 Repeat on the other side.

5 Repeat this step several times.

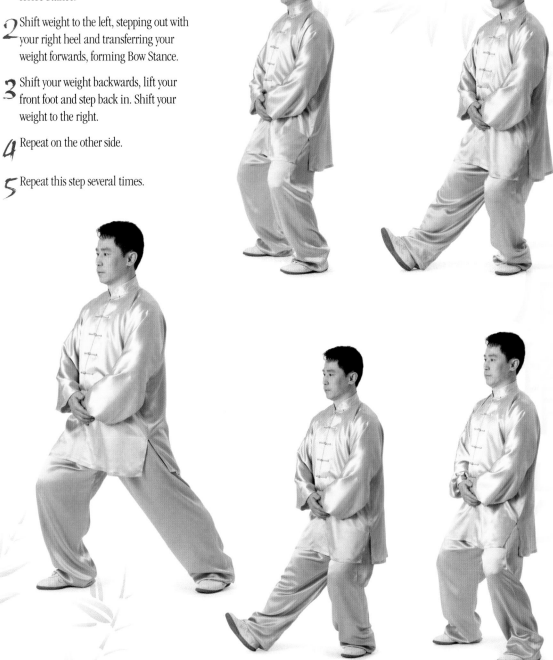

STEPPING OUT TO THE CORNER
斜，上步

1 For the purpose of learning, start in Horse Stance.

2 Shift your weight to the right, turn your body leftwards, step out to the corner with your left heel and transfer weight forwards, forming Bow Stance.

3 Shift your weight backwards and pivot the left toes in.

4 Shift your weight to the left while pivoting your right heel in.

5 Repeat on the other side.

6 Repeat this step several times.

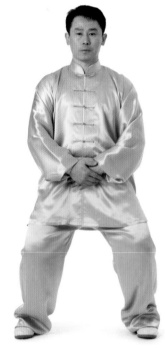
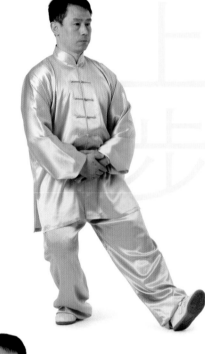
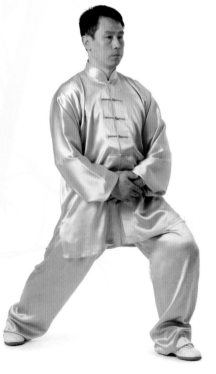
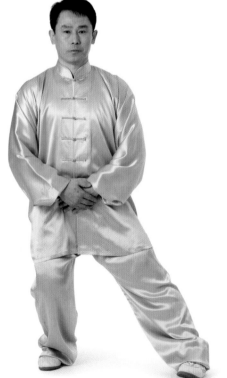

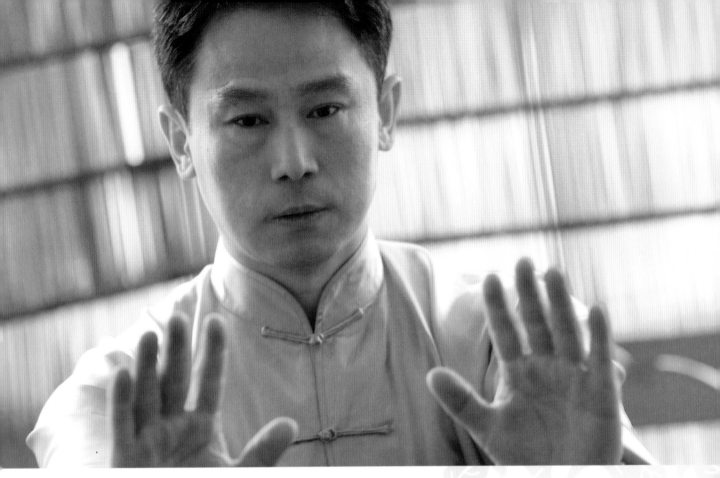

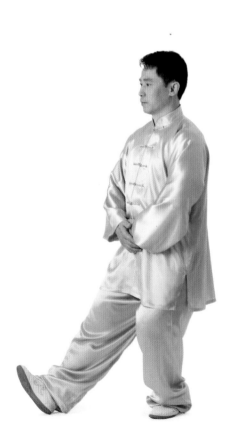

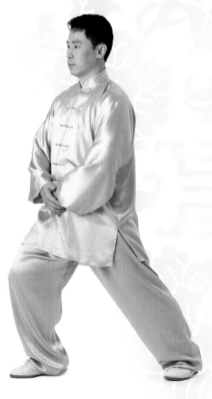

Tai Chi 8 Form

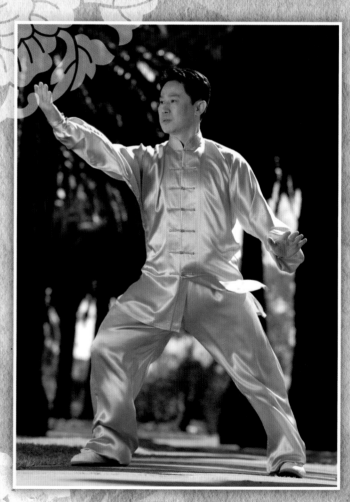

This is a basic Yang-style Tai Chi form consisting of eight Tai Chi movements. It is a good foundation for grasping the basics of Yang-style Tai Chi. As you become more familiar with this form, practise it regularly to enjoy its relaxing effect.

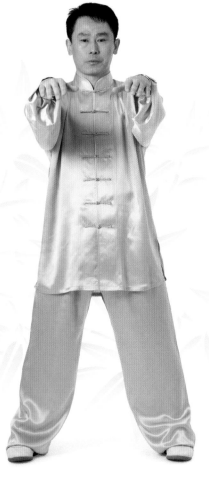

RAISING HANDS　起式

1 Stand with your feet apart and focus on using the Ba Hui pressure point to lead your head upwards.

2 Raise your hands to shoulder width and shoulder height.

3 Drop your elbows and press your palms down, bending your knees at the same time, as in Horse Stance.

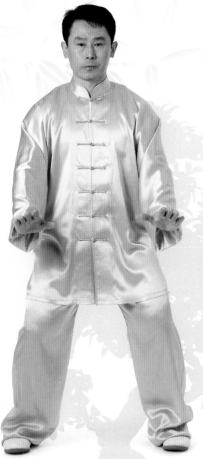

Repulse Monkey　倒攆猴

1 Turn your body to the right, separate both hands, and raise them to shoulder height with palms up.

2 Bend your right elbow, pushing forwards over your front hand.

3 Turn your body to the left and raise your left hand up to shoulder height with your palm up.

4 Bend your left elbow and push forwards over your front hand.

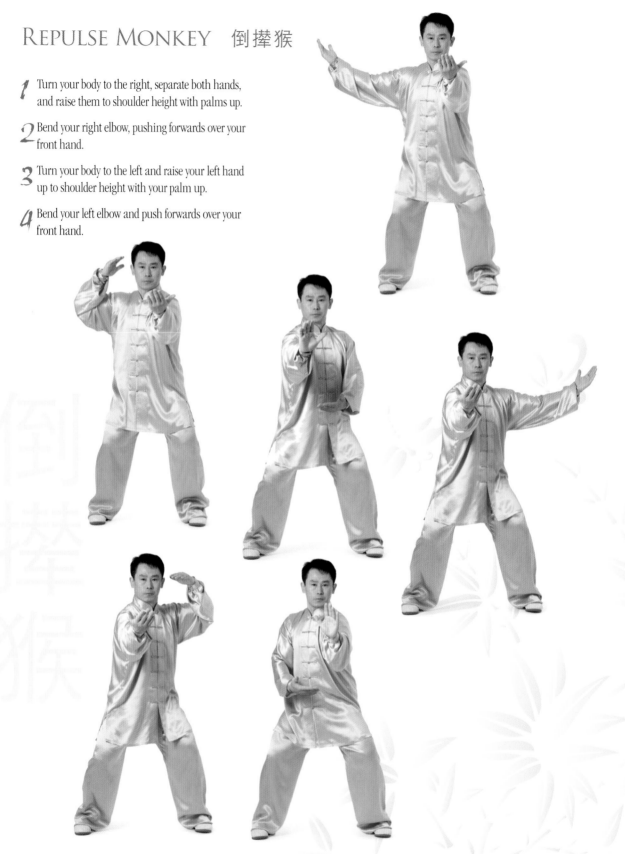

BRUSH KNEE　搂膝拗步

1 Block your left hand by pushing to the right and
continue to raise your right hand up to shoulder
height while transferring your weight to the right.

2 Turn your body and step to the corner with your
left heel. At the same time, lower your left arm and
bend your right elbow.

3 Block your left arm to the side by sweeping across
to the left side over the knee to front of hip, and
push with your right hand while transferring your
weight forwards, forming Bow Stance.

4 Repeat on the other side.

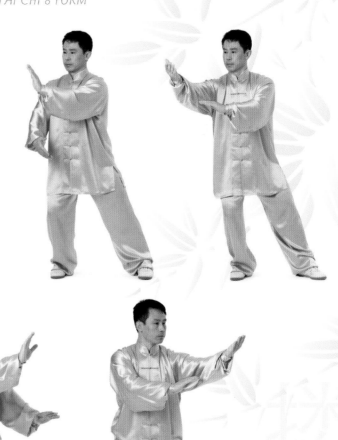

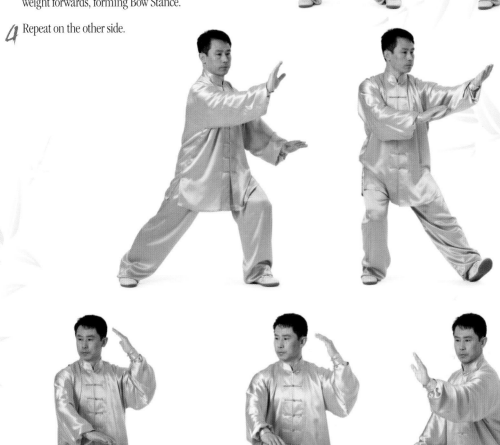

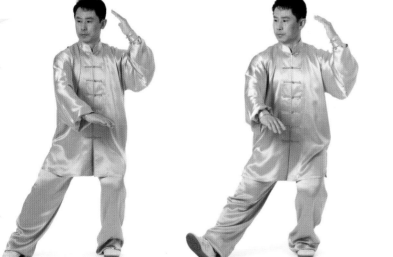

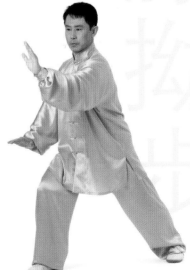

PARTING THE HORSE'S MANE
野马分鬃

1 Transfer your weight leftwards and open your left arm while pivoting your right toes in.

2 Transfer your weight to the right, arms in 'holding the ball' with your right hand on top.

3 Step to the left corner, while extending left arm out.

4 Separate both arms (bottom arm going up and forwards, top arm going down and backwards) and transfer your weight forwards, forming Bow Stance.

5 Repeat on the other side.

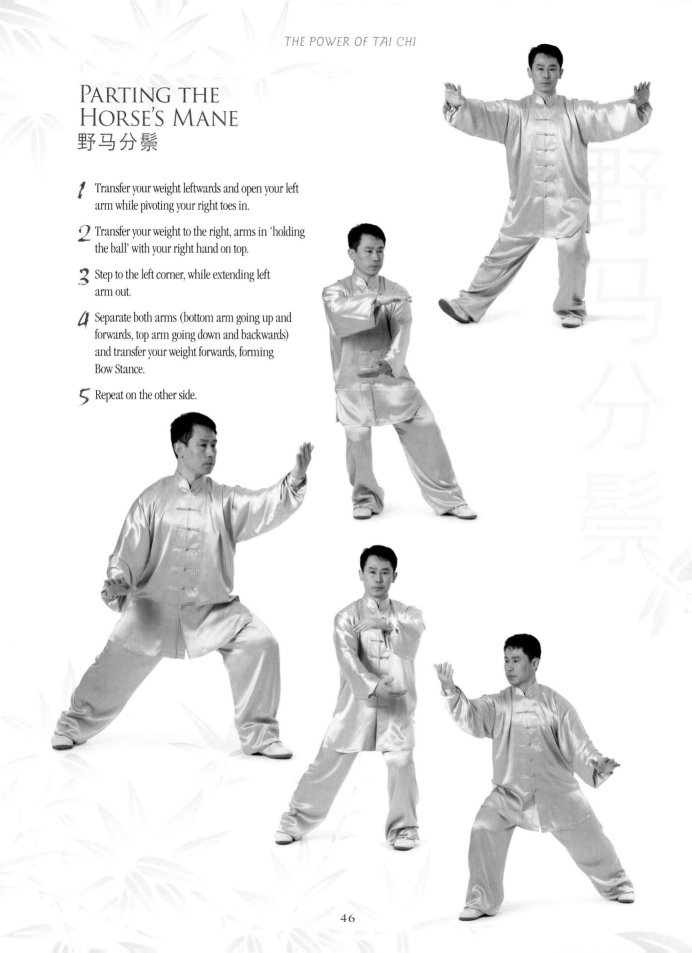

CLOUD HANDS (WITHOUT STEPPING) 云手

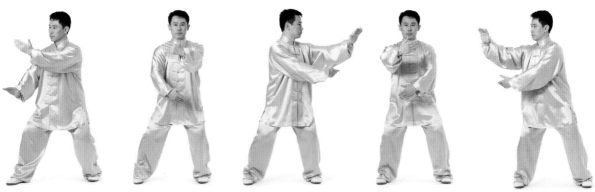

1 Press right hand to hip height, bring left hand up to shoulder height, while shifting weight backwards.

2 Turn both palms in, right toes step in to shoulder width and turn your body to the left.

3 Press your left hand down to the side while bringing your right hand up to shoulder height.

4 Repeat on the other side.

5 Repeat twice more on both sides.

GOLDEN ROOSTER STANDS ON ONE LEG 金鸡独立

1 Lower both arms and pull towards left.

2 Turn left palm face down, while pivoting left toes open, right hand following to the front.

3 Lift your right hand and right knee forwards.

4 Step your right foot down and shift your weight to the right while pressing right hand down to the side.

5 Repeat on the other side.

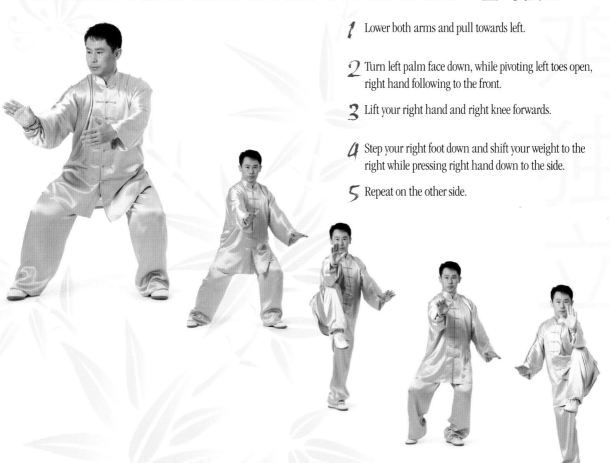

JADE LADY 玉女穿梭

1 Step your left foot down, arms 'holding a ball' with left arm on top. Shift your weight to the left.

2 Step out to the corner with your right heel, blocking to the same direction with your outer right forearm.

3 Continue to block upwards with outer right forearm, and push forward with your left hand, forming Bow Stance.

4 Transfer your weight backwards while relaxing your arms.

5 Transfer weight back, pivot right toes in and step back. Drop left arm to form 'holding a ball', with right arm on top.

6 Repeat on the other side.

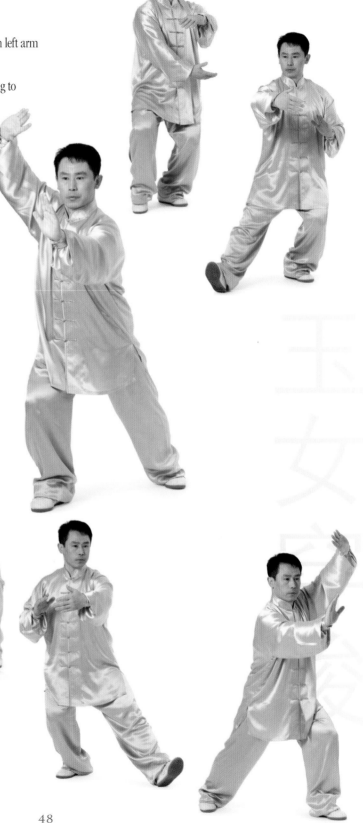

PRESS AND PUSH   捋挤式

1 Transfer your weight backwards while relaxing your arms in front at shoulder height, and pivot left toes in.

2 Step your left foot back in and press your hands down.

3 Shift your weight to the left, raise both hands up to shoulder height.

4 Cross your hands in front of your chest and step out with your right heel at the same time.

5 Press forwards while shifting your weight to form Bow Stance.

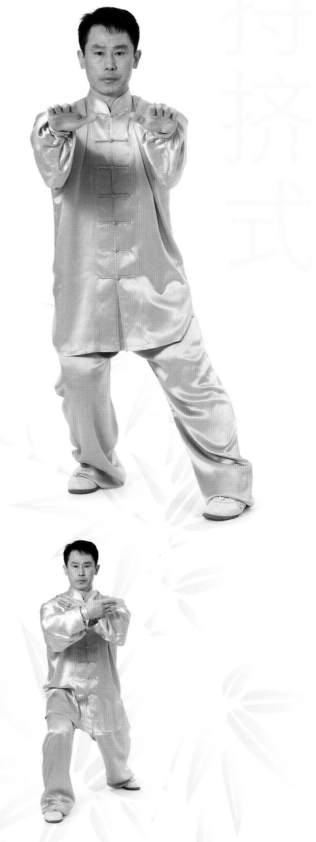

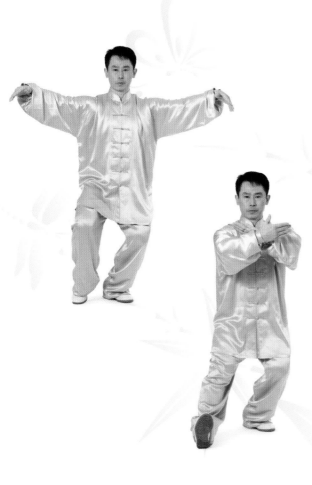

6 Separate your hands to shoulder width.

7 Pull your hands back towards your chest in a circular motion while shifting your weight backwards. At the same time, pivot your front toes up.

8 Continuing the circular motion, push your hands down, forwards and up to the front at chest height while shifting your weight forwards to form Bow Stance.

9 Repeat on the other side.

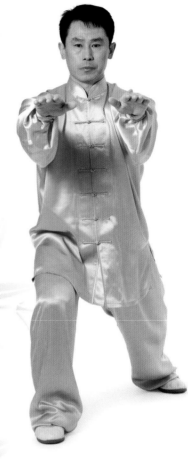

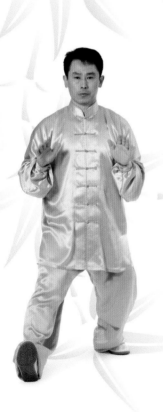

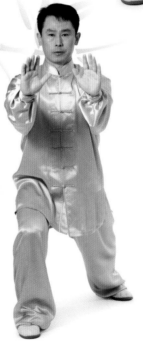

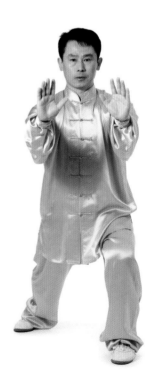

CROSS HANDS 十字手

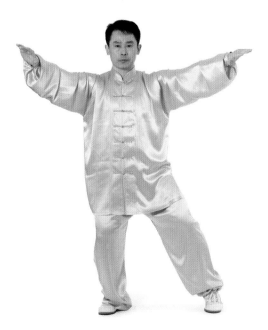

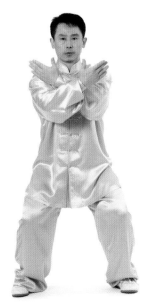

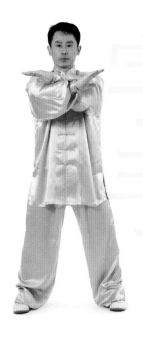

1 Step your left foot back in to shoulder width, separating your hands down to the side and shifting your weight to the left.

2 Cross your arms in front of your chest and pivot your right toes to the front. Adjust your weight to the centre of your body, knees remaining slightly bent as in Horse Stance.

3 Slowly straighten legs and turn palms down.

CLOSING

1 Uncross your arms, separating them down to relax beside your body.

2 Shift your weight to the right, and step your left foot in.

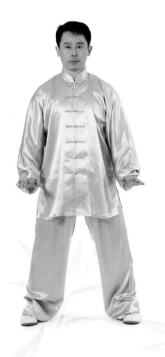

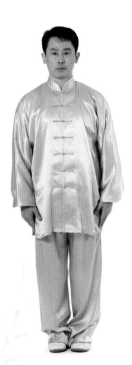

COOLING DOWN EXERCISES

It is beneficial to finish each session with some cooling down exercises, which help to relieve any muscular or joint discomfort, like tightness or fatigue, that might have occurred during the exercises. It also returns the qi to the origin (Lower Dan Tian).

RELAXATION MASSAGE 放松按摩

1 Tuck your thumbs under your index fingers.

2 Pat your lower back using the area of your hand indicated.

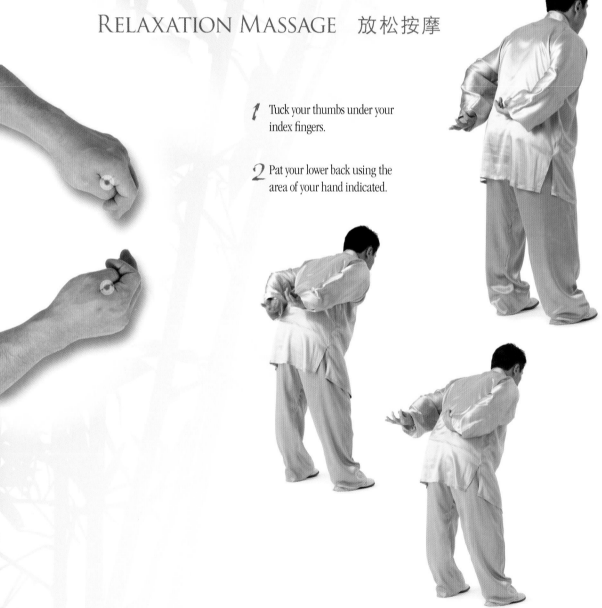

3 Continue patting down to your buttocks, and the backs, sides and fronts of your thighs.

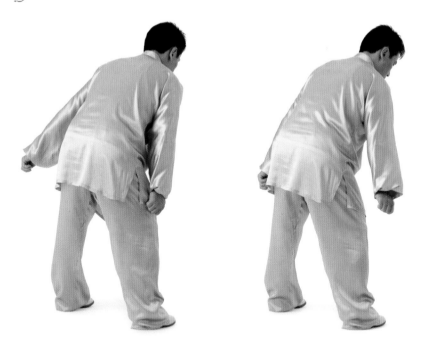

4 Place your hands over your knees and massage in a circular motion.

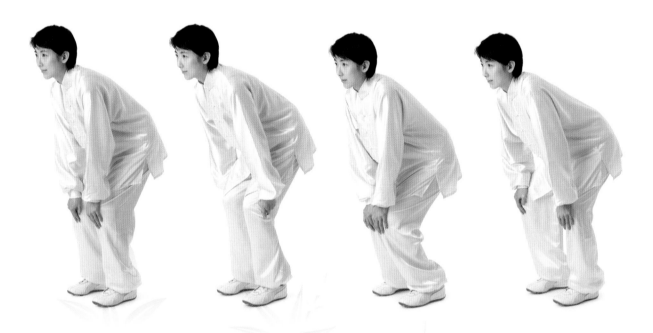

5 Leaving your hands on your knees, bend your knees, and use your hands to push down while slowly standing up.

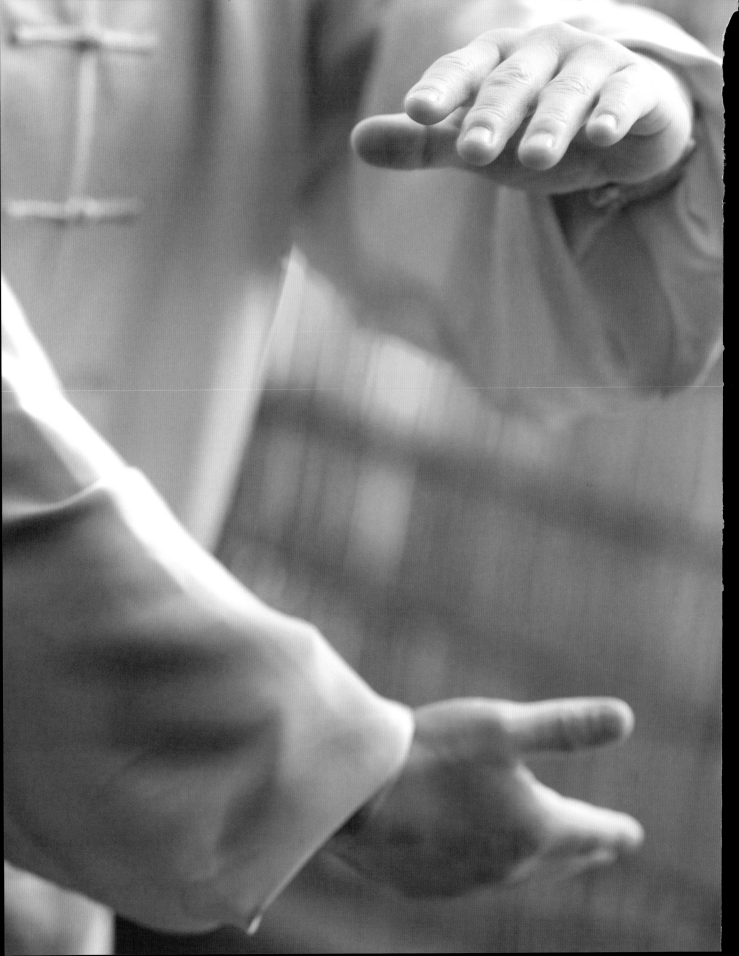

RETURNING QI TO THE ORIGIN 引气归元

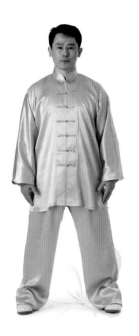
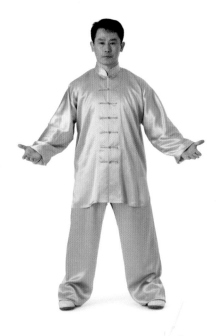

1 Breathe in. Raise your arms up from your sides, palms facing up.

2 Breathe out. When your arms reach the top, bend your elbows slightly, lowering your arms and pressing your palms down in front of your body.

3 Repeat 2–3 times.

4 After pressing your palms down in front of your body, cross them over the Lower Dan Tian (women should have their left hand on top, men their right hand on top). The Lao Gong pressure points of the palms will be aligned with the Lower Dan Tian. Keep tongue touching the palate of the mouth and maintain this position for a few minutes or as long as comfortable.

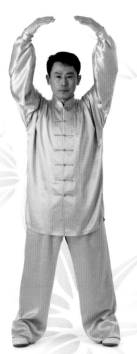
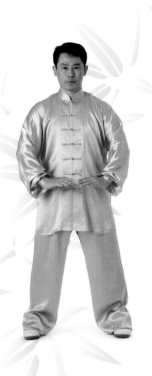
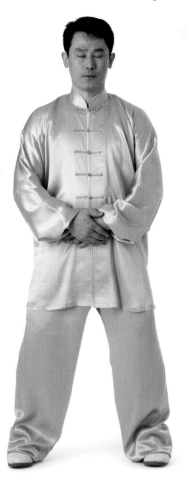

Tai Chi Standing Meditation

太极桩

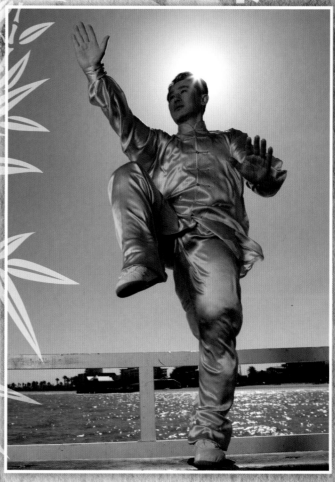

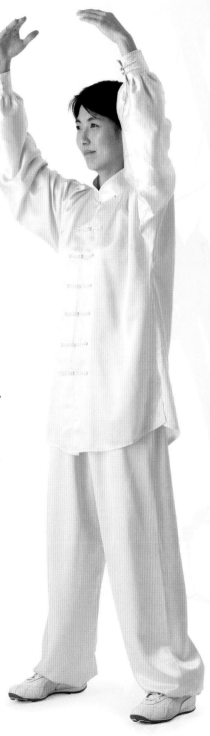

Tai Chi standing meditation is excellent for cultivating qi, in particular the Dan Tian qi, opening up the body's energy channels, maintaining proper posture and helping the practitioner become more grounded. The beauty of this meditation is that it can be done any time. Regular practice can help further understanding of one's inner qi, increase one's internal or core strength, in particular the ward-off strength, and help the smooth flow of qi in the body. Ward-off strength is an important internal strength often used in Tai Chi Pushing Hands and martial applications. In ward-off, internal energy is channelled to the forearms as a defence mechanism.

There are a couple of traditional Tai Chi sayings about standing meditation:

- 'standing meditation cures a hundred illnesses.'
  站桩治百病
- 'focus on Dan Tian to train the inner strength; the strength can be heard in the practitioner's explosion of breath.'
  拿住丹田练内功，哼哈二气妙无穷

MEDITATIVE SEQUENCE

1   Standing with feet apart, raise your hands to shoulder height.

2   Drop your elbows and press your palms down, bending your knees slightly at the same time, as in Horse Stance.

3   Turn your palms to face your lower abdomen, aligning the Lao Gong pressure point to the Lower Dan Tian.

4   Contract/hold the pelvic floor muscles while maintaining this posture for as long as possible and as is comfortable.

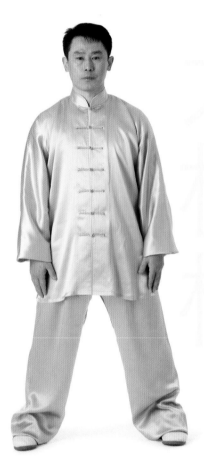

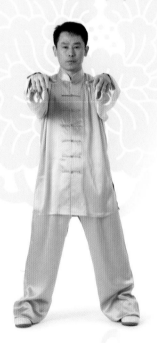

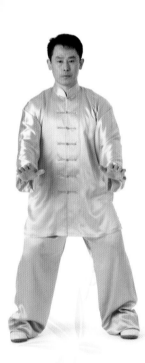

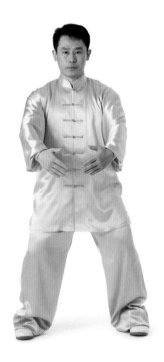

5 Slowly straighten your knees. Gently press your palms towards the Lower Dan Tian and relax your hands to the side while turning your palms to face up.

6 While breathing in, raise your arms up from your sides over your head.

7 While breathing out, relax your elbows by bending slightly, lowering your arms and pressing your palms down in front of your body and relax your hands to the side.

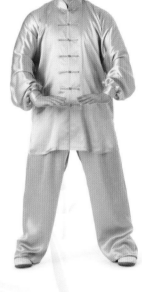

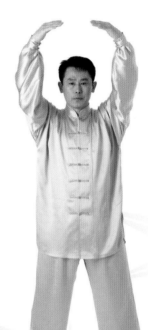

Notes

1 During this standing meditation, you should keep your tongue gently touching the top of your mouth's palate. This will help connect the Governor and Conception Meridians, helping the flow of qi. It also generates saliva, which is considered an important body fluid in Chinese medicine, nourishing the organs, reducing stress and helping to centre your mind.

2 When in this posture, try to consciously push the Ming Men pressure point backwards. This will sink the qi down to the Lower Dan Tian and stretch the spine, thus aiding the smooth flow of qi.

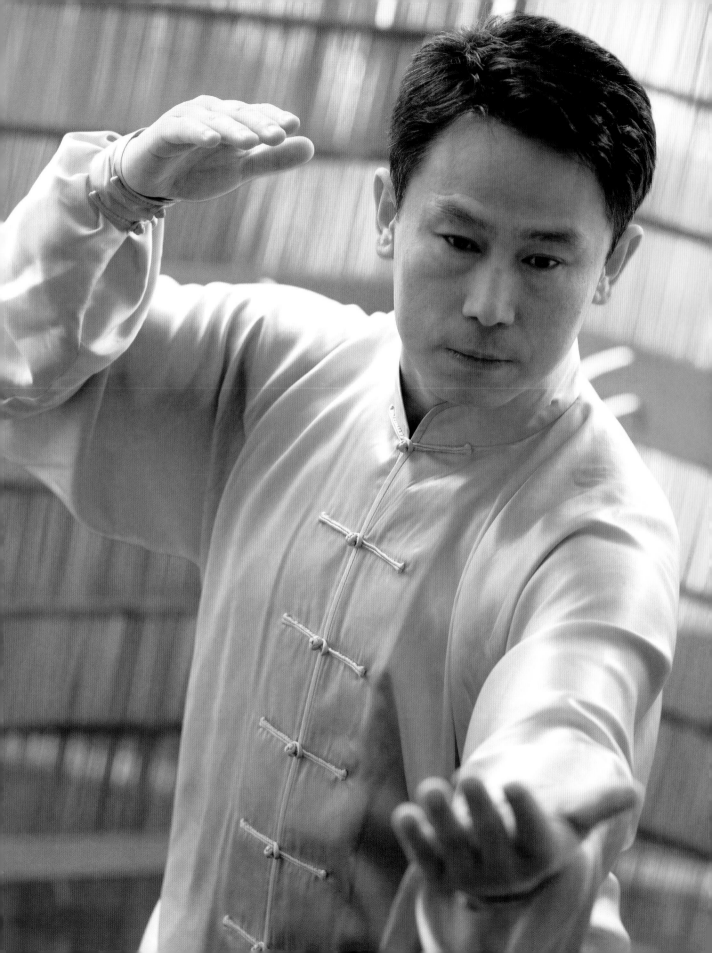

CONCLUSION

The aim of this book was to introduce the principles of Tai Chi, and help you establish some foundation skills for further Tai Chi practice. You can keep this book as a handy Tai Chi reference for the future.

You are now equipped with a basic understanding and the foundation skills of Tai Chi. More advanced training may involve pushing hands, martial applications, or training with equipment such as aids and weapons, and learning the different styles of Tai Chi. Whether or not you choose to progress to more advanced Tai Chi practice, the skills and knowledge you have gained from this book can be used to help improve and maintain your health and wellbeing for the rest of your life! Thank you for letting us share the first steps of your Tai Chi journey – we hope to share more of the treasure of Tai Chi with you in the future.

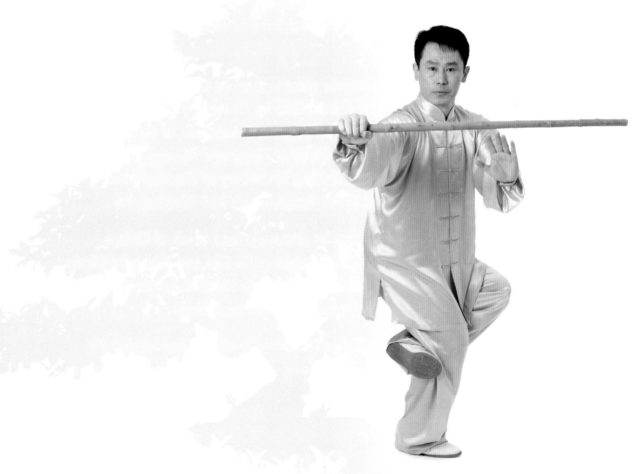

ABOUT THE AUTHOR

Master Shao Zhao-Ming was influenced by his family and started Chinese martial arts (Kung Fu-Wushu) at the early age of five with Grandmaster Zhang Tong, China's renowned Tai Chi, BaGua and Xing Yi master.

He sustained a serious back injury at the age of 15 that threatened to end his martial arts career. However, by practising two hours of Qi Gong meditation training every day, he was able to make a full recovery. This gave him a great understanding and insight into the concept of qi and Dan Tian. He went on to become the National Open Champion of China Kung Fu-Wushu (martial arts) in 1989 and 1990.

In the field of martial arts, Master Shao's Broadsword and Cudgel routines were selected for the textbook used by universities and institutes of sport in China. Dedication to his studies and training has resulted in his attainment of 'Wu Ying', the highest level of Kung Fu-Wushu and Tai Chi awarded by the Sports Commission of China.

Traditional Chinese medicine and Chinese martial arts are closely related and Master Shao has studied and graduated from Beijing University of Traditional Chinese Medicine and Beijing University of Physical Education. In the field of Chinese medicine, he is the author of *The Study of Therapeutic Massage for Injury*, which is now a textbook and subject at Beijing University of Physical Education. He has attained the Master of Medicine in Acupuncture and Moxibustion.

Due to his achievements and knowledge, he was appointed coach of China's prestigious Beijing University of Physical Education Tai Chi and Kung Fu-Wushu team. He is the vice president of The Martial Arts and Medical Research Institute of the Traditional Chinese Medicine Association (Beijing, China).

He now has a clinical practice in traditional Chinese medicine and teaches the Chinese martial arts of Tai Chi, Qi Gong, Kung Fu-Wushu and Bagua Zhang at the Tai Chi Kung Fu Institute in Melbourne.

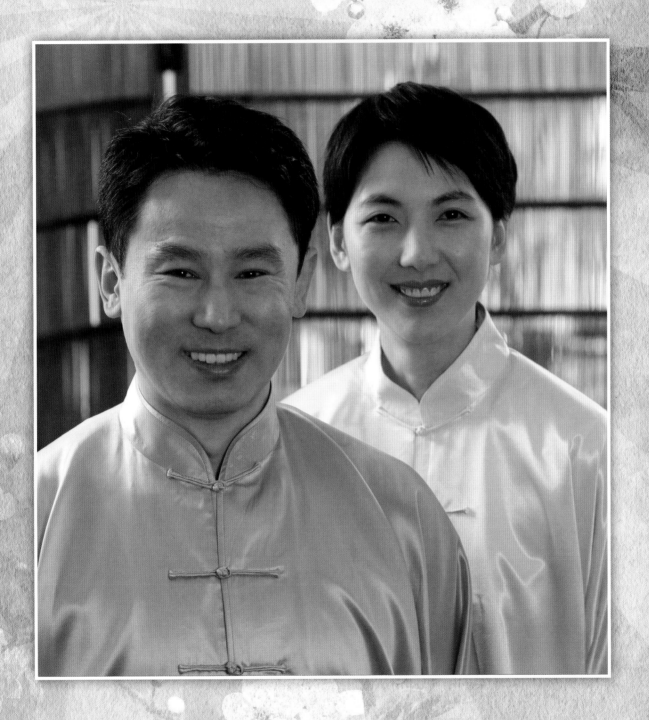

ACKNOWLEDGEMENTS

The priceless gifts of knowledge in Chinese martial arts, Tai Chi and Qi Gong have been generously shared with me by teachers to whom I am forever grateful:

- **Grandmaster Zhang Tong (1917–2005)**
  Renowned Grandmaster of Chinese martial arts and Tai Chi. My master and an inspiration who dedicated his whole life to the teaching and promotion of Chinese martial arts and Tai Chi.

- **Professor Li Yong Chang**
  Expert and ideologist in Chinese medicine and Qi Gong. Professor Li has been an inspirational teacher/master to me in the journey of Chinese medicine and Qi Gong. He is the founder and president of the Chinese Martial Arts Medicine Association.

- **Grandmaster Bai Wen Xiang**
  Dedicated martial arts teacher who has been an important influence in my career.

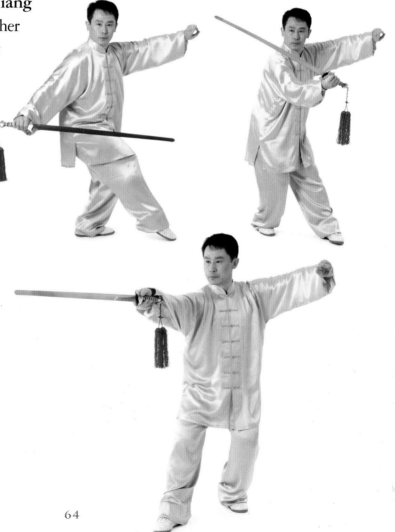

So precious are these gifts that they can only be fully appreciated when shared with all who have the fortune to come across them. As such, it is a part of my life's journey to spread and promote Tai Chi, and the Chinese healing and martial arts. It is with joy that my wife Ching shares this passion and joins me on this journey.